CULTIVATING MUSHROOM SIMPLIFIED

COMPLTE GUIDE ON HOW TO MAKE MUSHROOMS AT HOME AND OTHER PLACES

KADIE WATSON

Table of Contents

CHAPTER ONE

How to Make Mushrooms

There are six popular types of mushrooms that can be grown in your own backyard:

What Is a Mushrooms

Spores give rise to the fleshy fungus known as the mushroom. Mushrooms can be found in a variety of dishes, from mushroom pizza to mushroom risotto to oyster mushroom sautée. Different parts of the fungus appear on dinner plates

depending on the type of mushroom. Only the mushroom cap is eaten in some cases. Mushroom mycelium (a network of thread-like filaments) serves as a binding agent in other cases, such as tempeh.

It is possible to cultivate and harvest fresh mushrooms in your own backyard or house if you shop at a grocery store or farmers market. Because mushrooms are fungi rather than plants, their growth is not the same as that of vegetables. Beginners can go from

mushroom spawn to a delicious mushroom crop in just a few weeks with careful attention to the right growing medium and temperature.

Everything tastes better when you grow it yourself. Mushrooms thrive in cool, dark, and moist conditions, unlike most other vegetables. Although mushrooms can be grown outside, the process can take up to three years if there are inconsistencies in the growing conditions. Growing them at home is best done in a dark basement or under a sink, away from direct sunlight. If you have a limited amount of space, you can grow mushrooms.

When growing mushrooms in an indoor environment, you'll need a different type of growing medium for each type of mushroom. It will explain how to grow white button mushrooms, which are actually the same species as cremini and portabello mushrooms.

PRIOR TO DEPARTURE:

Mushrooms are grown in a different manner than most other vegetables. It's critical that we define a few key terms before moving on to discuss how plants grow.

Most plants are grown from seed, but mushrooms and other fungi are grown from spores.

Mycelium, a white, root-like substance, forms when mushroom spores are mixed with soil or another growing medium.

Mycelium can grow on a substrate called a mushroom substrate. compost and manure are ideal substrates for growing white button mushrooms.

Mycelium grows on a substrate known as mushroom spawn.

PRIOR TO DEPARTURE:

Mushrooms are grown in a different manner than most other vegetables. Before we get into the specifics of the growing process, we need to define a few key terms.

Mushrooms and other fungi are grown from spores, unlike most plants.

Mycelium, a white, root-like substance, forms when mushroom spores are mixed with soil or another growing medium.

Mycelium can grow on a substrate called a mushroom substrate. compost and manure are ideal substrates for growing white button mushrooms.

Mycelium grows on a substrate known as mushroom spawn

CHAPTER TWO

How to Grow 6 Popular Mushrooms at Home

Many types of edible mushrooms are popular with home growers. Commercial mushroom farms can easily produce all of these species, but they are all suitable for home cultivation.

Japanese cuisine is famous for its use of shiitake mushrooms, a type of mushroom. Mushrooms known as shiitake are known for their meaty texture and umami flavor. As a vegetable, they can be sautéed or stir-fried or roasted, served as a pizza topping, or added to soup.

Oyster mushrooms have a mild and sweet flavor and are white to light brown in color. For stir-fries and soups, oyster mushrooms are a common ingredient in Chinese cuisine.

Sliced white button mushrooms are a common ingredient on pizzas and pasta dishes.

Fruit of the tooth fungus Lion's mane mushroom is bulbous at first but eventually becomes round. A lion's mane or a large beard can be seen in mature organisms.

Popular in Italian cuisine, this mushroom is dense and hearty. In portobello mushroom burgers, portobello mushrooms are used as a meat substitute.

A hen-of-the-woods mushroom, maitake mushrooms can be grown in captivity as well as in the wild. The soft overlapping caps of these mushrooms are sold in clusters. This mushroom is found in the northwestern United States and Japan and has an earthy aroma.

Mushrooms: How to Grow Them

Oyster mushrooms, shiitake mushrooms, and nearly any other mushroom species can be grown successfully if the right conditions are provided.

Grow mushrooms in the house. Despite the fact that you can grow mushrooms in your garden, it is much easier to cultivate a large mushroom harvest indoors. Mushrooms can grow without sunlight because they are fungi. In order to thrive, they require a constant supply of cool, moist air, which can be easily controlled indoors. As long as you have an area that isn't too hot (like your basement or garage), you can grow mushrooms. Fifty-five to sixty degrees Fahrenheit is the ideal temperature range for growing plants.

Assemble a suitable growing medium. 2. 2. Mushrooms, in contrast to most plants, do not thrive in potting soil. If you're looking for shiitake mushrooms, you'll want to use wood chips or hardwood sawdust; composted manure, straw, or coffee grounds are also good options (also good for oyster mushrooms). In a container at least six inches deep, place your growing medium (also known as a substrate). As a result, mushroom mycelium can grow unhindered.

Take your mushrooms and inoculate them. Mushrooms can be grown in a variety of ways. Mushroom spores (like plant seeds) or mushroom spawn can be planted (the equivalent of plant seedlings). For the first harvest, beginners should use mushroom spawn and then move on to spores. Unlike other organisms, you don't have to press these into their substrate. Add a quarter-inch of substrate on top of them and sprinkle them on top.

To get the mushrooms growing, keep the spawns warm. You can speed up the growth of your mushrooms by keeping them at a temperature of seventy degrees Fahrenheit for the first few days of their development. To provide even more warmth, place a heating pad under the container.

Keep your crops well watered, but not drenched. Moisture is essential to the growth of mushrooms, but soaking wet mushrooms do not thrive. Using a spray bottle, mist your crops from time to time, but don't let the growing medium become soggy. Mushroom growers sometimes use a moist cloth or an open plastic bag to keep moisture in the container.

After a few weeks, it's time to gather your mushrooms. Fruiting is the term used to describe the process of mushrooms sprouting. As a general rule, this will happen within three to four weeks. The crop will start out as tiny mushrooms and quickly grow into something substantial. When a mushroom's cap is fully open and begins to separate from the stem, it is ripe. To keep the cycle going, you can replenish the growing medium with fresh mushroom spawn.

Consume newly harvested mushrooms within a few days. The shelf life of fresh mushrooms is only a few days. If you don't plan on using them right away, consider freezing them instead. In order to feed the next generation of mushroom spawn or spores, old mushrooms can be composted.

CHAPTER THREE

A guide to mushroom cultivation.

Mushrooms are best grown in a climate-controlled environment, such as a greenhouse. There are many options for growing mushrooms in the shade, such as a shed, garage, cold frame, or cellar. Mushrooms prefer temperatures between 10°C and 20°C for optimum growth. Mushrooms can be grown in beds, on compost heaps and logs, all of which should be kept out of the direct sunlight.

Mushrooms can be grown in beds or containers.

Mushrooms require a moist, fertile, and nutrient-rich growing medium. You can buy horse manure from your local garden center or nearby stables for mushroom cultivation. Fresh manure should be placed in a heap and forked over every couple of days for a week to ensure that it is thoroughly mixed and allowed time to cool and settle.

The growing medium should be kept damp. Cover the spawn with damp newspaper and spread it out to a depth of 5-8cm. Take off the newspaper after a few weeks, and cover the white thread-like mycelium with a 2-3cm layer of garden soil or compost mixed with a 50/50 mixture of lime. Use a hose with a spray attachment or a watering can with a fine rose to water as needed to keep this evenly moist. After a few weeks of sowing, mushrooms should begin to appear.

Mushrooms can be grown on logs.

Mushroom log kit teaches you how to cultivate mushrooms.

Once the dowels are inserted into the logs, growing mushrooms on logs is a cinch. Logs are required, but you don't have to supply or drill them for yourself. The wood should be healthy and preferably not from a conifer. Dowels should be inserted no more than six weeks after the logs have been freshly cut. Oak, beech, hornbeam, chestnut, hazel, birch, maple, and holly are some of the best woods to use in furniture construction and carving. Logs should be 45-60cm long with a diameter of 10-15cm.

Drill holes every 15cm and every 8cm along the length of the log. The impregnated dowels should be inserted completely into the holes. Some kits include sealing wax, so use it if instructed. A shady spot, under trees or shrubs, with one end on the ground and the other propped up is ideal. It can take up to 18 months for mushrooms to grow.

Oyster mushrooms can be grown in a variety of ways.

Oyster mushroom spawn and straw are all you need to get started. Make sure the straw is thoroughly wet by soaking it overnight in water and removing any excess water. Make a polythene bag out of a bin liner by mixing the mushroom spawn with the damp straw. In a damp, sheltered location between 20-25oC, such as near your compost heap, seal and leave for six weeks. The mushroom spawn will grow into the straw as it decomposes, colonizing it.

Oyster mushrooms can be grown in straw by Monty Don.

Oyster mushroom spores will have colonized the straw in the plastic bag within six weeks of planting them. Your greenhouse is a good place to keep the bags in an area that is both light and moist. Oyster mushrooms can grow through the bag's slits.

A visit from Monty Don to see how his oyster mushrooms are doing:

You should check the bag after two weeks to see if oyster mushrooms have grown inside of it. Mushrooms can be expected to grow on the straw for at least a week more.

Mushroom buying advice

Some vegetable seed companies, as well as

specialized mushroom suppliers, offer spawn and dowels for growing mushrooms via mail order.

Choose the appropriate mushroom kit for your requirements and available space. Your mushrooms' success depends on providing them with the ideal conditions.

Forage sources in the area

- Spectacular mushrooms

- Suttons

THE END

www.ingramcontent.com/pod-product-compliance
Lightning Source LLC
LaVergne TN
LVHW012034160826
845678LV00013B/2592

* 9 7 9 8 8 4 5 8 5 0 4 6 1 *